I0062516

Maca (The Medicinal Plant of the Inkas)

How To Improve Your Sex Drive, Sperm Quality and women dillodo with Maca, Control Cancer, Virility, Depression and Erectile Dysfunction. (Maca For Pregnancy, Menopause Symptoms, Athletic Performance)

Dionisia Onio

Copyright © 2022 by Dionisia Onio.

All rights reserved. No part of this publication may be reproduced, distributed, or transmitted in any form or by any means, including photocopying, recording, or other electronic or mechanical methods, without the prior written permission of the publisher, except in the case of brief quotations embodied in critical reviews and certain other non-commercial uses permitted by copyright law.

Table of Contents

INTRODUCTION

Firstly, I need to congratulate you for getting a copy of this book. I believe that you will be full of joy after reading Maca (The Medicinal Plant of The Inkas) and do not forget to recommend the book for your friends and family.

Imagine a plant, a plain tuber, that looks like a radish, that grows at an altitude of 4000 meters, that survives extreme heat, cold, severe weather and a thin atmosphere and which at the same time stores strength, vitamins, trace elements and mineral nutrients. The Inkas had already used maca root from the Andean high plateaus as food and as medicine. Peter Carl Simons, a health expert, shows how this unremarkable plant can still be used as part of a therapy. The field of application includes: cancer therapy, erectile dysfunction, depression, premature birth and female fertility, anaemia, endocrine disorder, and many other. The maca root is also known in the context of anti-aging therapy.

CHAPTER 1

What Is Maca?

Maca is a nutritionally dense super food that has been used for hundreds of years. Maca is unique in that it affects men and women differently. In this book i will detail how and why to apply this first-rate food.

Before i outline the foremost advantages of Maca for women, we want to point out that there are numerous types of Maca available. Maca for women the different forms/types of maca have various effects and work better for helping specific health conditions. I indicate which Maca is best for each of the benefits indexed below.

Maca Nutrition

Maca root powder is an excellent source of protein, fiber and numerous vitamins and minerals, such as vitamin C, copper and iron. It also contains over 20 amino acids — inclusive of all eight essential amino acids — and lots of health-promoting *phytonutrients*.

One ounce (or about 2 tablespoons) of maca powder contains approximately:

- 91 energies

- 20 grams carbohydrates

- 4 grams protein

- 1-gram fats

- 2 grams dietary fiber

- 79.8 milligrams vitamin C (133 percent DV)

- 1.7 milligrams copper (84 percent DV)

- 4.1 milligrams iron (23 percent DV)

- 560 milligrams potassium (16 percentage DV)

- 0.3 milligram diet b6 (16 percent DV)

- 0.2 milligram manganese (11 percentage DV)

- 1.6 milligrams niacin (8 percent DV)

- 70 milligrams calcium (7 percent DV)

- 0.1milligram riboflavin (6 percentage DV)

Maca Nutrition Fact

In general Maca is rich in amino acids, phytonutrients, fatty acids, diet and minerals. According to nutritional research Maca contains

1. **59% carbohydrates** – Maca is rich in quality carbs, which, combined with its alkaloids and other nutrients make it an amazing choice for sustained energy.

2. **10.2% protein** – Maca is loaded with

bio-available plant protein that is easy for the body to assimilate

3. **8.5% fiber** – Maca contains quite high levels of cellulose and lignan, both of which stimulate intestinal function. Fiber is a key factor to a healthy digestive and elimination system.

4. **Essential Amino Acids:** Maca contains nearly all of them. These drive many cellular functions in the body including sexual and fertility functions.

- Aspartic Acid – 97 mg/1 g protein

- Glutamic Acid – 156 mg/1 g protein

- Serine – 50 mg/1 g protein

- Histidine – 22 mg/1 g protein

- Glycine – 68 mg/1 g protein

- Arginine – 99.4 mg/ 1 g protein

- Threonine – 33 mg/1 g protein

- Alanine – 63 mg/1 g protein

- Tyrosine – 31 mg/1 g protein

- Phenylalanine – 55 mg/1 g protein

- Valine – 79 mg/1 g protein

- Methionine- 28 mg/1 g protein

- Isoleucine – 47 mg/1 g protein

- Leucine – 91 mg/1 g protein

- Lysine – 55 mg/1 g protein

- Ho- proline- 26 mg/1 g protein

- Proline – .5mg/1 g protein

- Sarcosine – .7mg/1 g protein

5. **Free fatty Acids:** 20 have been discovered in Maca. These also work to support cellular function. Saturated acids account for 40% and Non-saturated about 55%. The most abundant fatty acids adding to Maca's nutritional value are linolenic acid,

palmitic acid, oleic acid and steric acid.

- C12-0 -lauric – 0.8%

- C13-1-7 trideconoic – 0.3%

- C13-zero tridecoanoic – 0.1%

- C14-0 myrstic – 1.4%

- C15-1-7 pentadecanoic – 0.5%

- C16-1-9 palmtoleic – 2.7%

- C16-0 palmitic – 23.8%

- C17-1-9 heptadecenoic – 1.5%

- C17-0 heptadecanoic – 1.8%

- C18-2-9-12 linoleic – 32.6%

- C18-1-9 oleic – 11.1%

- C18-0 steric – 6.7%

- C19-1-11 nonadecenoic – 1.3%

- C19-0 – nonadecanoic – 0.4%

- C20-1-15 eisosenoic – 2.3%

- C22-0 behanic 2.0

- C24-1-15 nervonic – 0.4%

- C-24-0 lignocenic – 0.4%

6. Vitamins:

- Thamin (B1) – 1mg/100g – helps the body convert carbohydrates into energy. Important for good heart, muscle and nervous system function

- Riboflavin (B2) - .76mg/100g – important for body growth and red blood cell production

- Ascorbic Acid (C) - – 3mg/100g – helps anti-oxidant activity

- Niacin 35mg/100g – supports healthy circulation

7. Major minerals

- Calcium – 450mg/100g – Maca incorporates a higher level of calcium than most milk. Calcium is crucial in bone development as well as for nerve and circulatory system health.

- Phosphorus - 220mg/100g – phosphorus is crucial for the hemostasis of calcium as well as for transmitting electrical stimuli for brain and muscle action.

- Magnesium – 104mg/100g – magnesium is essential for the synthesis of protein and for muscle and nerve pastime. Crucial for coronary heart fitness.

- Potassium – 1500mg/100g – potassium works within the cells to help control and maintain healthy osmosis.

- Sodium 25mg/100g – together with potassium can support tremendous circulation

8. Minor minerals

- Copper – 5mg/100g – supports enzyme health.

- Zinc – 12mg/100g – Helps in clarity of idea and intellectual function

- Manganese – 8mg/100g – supports healthy growth

- Iron – 25mg/100g – important component of hemoglobin. Supports health muscle growth.

- Selenium – 20mg/100g – protects cells against free radicals.

- Boron – 5mg/100g – supports proper metabolism.

9. **Sterols** – with regular use sterols may have a positive impact on lowering blood cholesterol. One recent study confirmed that ingesting 1.8 to 2.8 grams of plant sterols and plant stanols per day over a period of 4 weeks to 3 months drastically lowered total cholesterol in participants by 7%-11%

- Brassicasterol – 9.1%

- Ergosterol – 13.6%

- Campesterol – 27.3%

- Ergostadienol – 4.5%

- Sitoserol – 46.5%

10. **Sugars:** Raw Maca contains 20g sugar per 100g and gelatinized Maca contains nearly 50g per 100g. These sugars are naturally occurring fruit sugars. However, diabetics ought to devour with caution. Liquid Maca extracts are suitable for diabetics.

11. **Glucosinolates:** Aromatic glucosinolates along with: benzyl glucosinolate, p-methoxybenzyl glucosinolate, fructose, glucose, benzyl isothiocyanate. In food-bearing plants, glucosinolates act as natural pesticides and are stored in the plant's cells, ready to be released upon tissue damage. Similarly, when consumed by people, the action of chewing releases the glucosinolates into the body, in where they're

transformed into bioactive compounds believed to have anticancer properties.

12. **Macaenes and macamides:** (Macaina 1, 2, 3, 4) these are polyunsaturated acids and their amides which are absolutely unique to Maca.

Beyond Maca Nutrition Facts – Maca As An Adaptogen

The Maca Nutrition facts indexed above show that Maca is a true dietary powerhouse and amazing daily food to put in your food plan (diet).

However, Maca root, like the Chinese herb ginseng, is also an adaptogen. Adaptogens are substances that raise the physical body's state of resistance to illnesses through physiological and emotional health improvements. This makes Maca a broad-based healer with many benefits able to support and rejuvenate overwhelmed, tired adrenal glands subsequently resulting in much greater energy, stamina, clarity of mind and spirit, and the capability to deal with stress.

One other important note is that scientists have also discovered that because of Maca's nutritional value, the food has the potential to regulate, support, and balance the hormonal systems of each man and women for most effective function. One of the very top-notch matters about Peruvian Maca root is that it is not "gender specific" and works equally properly for both women and men.

Maca And Weight Loss

Maca is a native Peruvian vegetable historically used as an aphrodisiac for women and men. Animal studies also show that it may help to improve endurance, according to the Memorial Sloan Kettering Cancer Centre. Maca, however, is not used for weight loss, and little evidence helps to support its use for this reason. Consult your health practitioner before adding any supplement on your daily routine.

Maca and Weight Gain

Maca may not be able to help you lose weight, however it might prevent weight gain, at least in postmenopausal rats. 2009 research published in the Journal of Hygiene Research investigated the effects of maca on body fat, as well as sexual hormones and bone metabolism, in female rats that had their ovaries taken out. The study found that the rats gain less weight when supplemented with maca. While this study indicates a few promises for maca in prevention of weight gain in women during menopause, human clinical trials are important to substantiate claims.

CHAPTER 2

Maca For Women's Fertility

Women have been using Maca powder to increase their chances of conceiving a child for over 2000 years. Clinical studies have proven that maca balances hormones which leads to regular ovulation. Additionally, Maca is a nutritional powerhouse that supports the optimal health needed to boost fertility. Red Maca has been shown to be the best maca for women seeking to boost their fertility.

Maca For Pregnancy

Maca is taken into consideration and generally safe to take during pregnancy stage. In reality, because of its high nutrient and mineral content, it could support healthy development. A 2-teaspoon serving of maca has 3 times more calcium than a glass of milk. Additionally, Black and Red Maca have been seen to increase bone density and strength. That said, if you have any worries about taking maca while you are pregnant, please seek advice from a competent medical expert.

Maca For Healthy Skin

Due to Maca's ability to help balance hormones, it frequently has a positive effect on pores and skin tone. This may include reducing hormone related pimples as well as improving skin elasticity. All maca powders which include cream colored maca works properly for this benefit.

Maca For Increased Libido

One of the biggest effects said by women taking proper dosages of Maca powder daily is a marked increase in sexual desire. Red Maca is the type of Maca that is highest in phytontutrients and, not surprisingly, is the maca of choice to enhance female libido.

Maca For Hot Flashes and Other Menopause Symptoms

Maca works very well to reduce all uncomfortable signs and symptoms of menopause and perimenopause inclusive of insomnia, mood swings and specifically hot flashes. This effect comes from maca's high-quality capacity to support healthy hormone balance. Maca does not contain hormones, but merely stimulates the body to balance the endocrine system. Red Maca is the best for women passing through this life transition.

Maca For Hair Growth

Because of Maca's brilliant hormone balancing properties in combination with its dense dietary content, the food is capable of stimulating hair growth in women who have thinning hair.

Maca For Reducing/Preventing Osteoperosis

Research have shown that Red and Black Maca were found to be the best at enhancing and protecting bone structure specifically in mice who had their ovaries removed. Other research have proven that maca increases bone strength and density.

Maca For Thyroid Health

Because of maca's hormone balancing properties, it has been suggested to have a positive effect on the health of the thyroid. Maca does contain iodine which affects the thyroid. If you have an iodine allergy you should avoid Maca.

Maca For Enhanced Curves

One of the more thrilling effects of Maca is that it can support the enhancement of female body shape. Maca works to balance estrogen levels, which can increase the size and shape of breasts. Additionally, considering the fact that Maca is extraordinarily anabolic (muscle building) it can increase the size of the buttocks, that which is of the body's largest muscle. If you want to get the most benefit for the latter, i recommend using Black Maca and also getting plenty of exercising aimed at increasing the glutes.

Maca For Women and Athletic Performance

Maca is exquisite for athletes. It builds muscle, it increases stamina, it boosts energy and it enhances recuperation time. Black Maca is my Maca of preference for athletes.

Maca For Reducing Depression

One of the lesser recognized benefits of Maca for women is for lowering depression. Maca works as a mood up-lifter because of its high nutrient content combined with its energizing properties. I've had numerous reports of positive emotional health resulting from continued use of Red Maca.

CHAPTER 3

Maca For Fertility

One of the most not unusual questions we get is from men and women who've heard about the use of Maca for fertility. Judging from these questions, there's a good misinformation out there regarding the way to use Maca to increase your chances of getting a baby. That's why i decided to put this comprehensive book together.

How The Use of Maca for Fertility Was Discovered

Maca (Lepidium meyenii) is a root vegetable that grows high in the Andes Mountains. It is in fact the world's highest growing food crop and has grown there naturally for thousands of years. The story of maca and fertility begins when Incan farmers observed how feeding maca roots to their farm animals made them more potent and healthier. With consistent maca feeding, the farmers also noticed that their animals had more and healthier babies.

It wasn't long after that people commenced the usage of maca to increase their own chances of conceiving. Natives of the Andes have long used maca for fertility purposes – and with good success. So much success that it was maca's fertility enhancing properties that first attracted North American and European researchers and doctors to start using it within the 1980s and 1990s.

How Maca Helps Both Male and Female Fertility

Maca is considered one of a few herbs that are believed to be "adaptogens." these special kinds of herbs adapt to a variety of conditions within a given body and help restore it to a healthy balance. Maca in particular works on the endocrine system to balance hormones in both males and females.

Clinical research, some of which are referenced below, have found that using of Black Maca boosts sperm count in men or even increases sperm activity. Similar studies show that female given Maca respond with increased regularity in cycles and less complicated ovulation. Some other result of taking maca is a marked increase in libido for both women and men.

Similarly to balance hormones taking maca also provides excellent nutritional support. Maca is rich in amino acids, phytonutrients, fatty acids, vitamin and minerals. Both women and men who are properly nourished substantially increase the likelihood of conceiving a healthy child.

How To Use Maca for Fertility

In case you decide to use maca for fertility purposes there are numerous things that you have to do and keep in mind in order to maximize your success.

- Use only high quality, fresh, certified organic maca powder. Unfortunately, there are many inferior products on the market that are made from chemically grown maca or from old maca roots that have lost their potency.

- Use the proper quantity of maca. Using Maca for fertility is considered to be a therapeutic utilization and therefore you need to take a therapeutic, always and often.

- Both partners should use maca. For optimum efficiency you and your companion have to be taking Maca. Maca comes with a number of other benefits, so it should to be easy to convince

33

him/her to do so.

- Women should consider using Red Maca for fertility. It is most nutritionally dense form of maca is and also the best for women fertility

- Men should use Black Maca for their fertility. Black Maca has been proven to increase sperm count and sperm motility

- Try cleansing and detox too. Completing an intensive cleansing program will help you get more out of Maca. That's because a good detox will cleanse your intestines and permit more nutrients to be absorbed by body.

- Do not forget getting this natural fertility resource. Similarly, to taking Maca there are many things you can do to increase your chances of a natural conception. The best resource I've seen is referred to as *Pregnancy Miracle*. It's jam pack with natural fertility strategies (along with taking Maca for fertility!)

Some Success Stories

Here are some couples who've reported having success using Maca for fertility.

"We tried a lot of things to get pregnant before we learned about Peruvian Maca in a book on natural fertility. My husband and i started taking it religiously after that. I got pregnant 6 months later and that I'm sure the Maca helped." *Jennifer and Ray Collins, Washington*

"I believe that Maca helped us to conceive naturally when traditional fertility treatments failed. I now have a happy & healthy baby." *Rachel. W, United Kingdom*

"My spouse (wife) and i were together for 7 years before we conceived. The only thing we did differently prior to that was to complete a round of serious detox and to start taking Maca. I'm convinced that Maca played an important part in getting pregnant." *Matt Leonard*

CHAPTER 4

Maca For Energy

The History and Tradition

We know that maca root has been used to boost energy for several thousand years. Although the first written connection with the simple root comes from 1553 in a chronicle of the Spanish conquest of the Andes, oral traditions confirm that the basis has long been valued as a dietary supplement, a fertility enhancer for each animal and humans and an energizer. Maca's potency was so valued to the inhabitants of high altitudes inside the Andes that it was regularly used as a currency for trade. In addition, warriors, both Incan and Spanish consume big amounts of maca root before going into warfare as a way to increase their energy, prowess and recovery time. In more recent times, maca's energy boosting properties are one of the major reasons it's become one of Peru's top agricultural exports.

What Does Science Say About Maca and Increased Energy?

Since the late 1990's many studies have been done on maca. A good number of them were focused on maca's potential to increase fertility and libido. There have simply been a few that have focused on maca and energy. However, the results have been impressive.

1. In 2009 five researchers from north Umbria University, Newcastle upon Tyne published a study carried out on athletes. One group of athletes was given maca powder for 14 days while another

group was given a placebo. At the end of the two weeks, they all finished a 40 km cycling course. When times were compared to previous bests on the same course, researchers discovered that the group taking maca notably reduced their times while the placebo group remained the same. The researchers concluded that the promising results suggest the need for longer and more clinical studies on maca for energy.

2. Another study in 2001 found that maca increased the energy and the sexual overall performance of male rats, making them both more able to reproduce and to sustain physical activities longer and more consistently.

3. A self-perception study performed in 2006 by G.E. Gonzalez confirmed that maca acted as an energizer in compared with placebo in otherwise healthy men.

4. Finally, a study from 2004 in Australia found out that maca powder, at a dosage of 3-5 grams per day, reduces psychological signs and symptoms, such as anxiety and depression, and lowers measures of sexual disorder in postmenopausal women independent of estrogenic and androgenic activity.

How Does Maca Work to Boost Energy?

Maca is very different from other types of energizers available in the market. It contains no caffeine, no processed sugar and no pharmaceutical energy enhancers. What that means is that maca boosts your energy in a balanced and sustained way and that it will never stresses your adrenal glands just like the aforementioned energy enhancers.

There Are Several Things Maca Does to Boost Your Energy:

1. Maca is a nutritional powerhouse. Maca root contains 10.5% protein, 8.5% fiber, 19 essential amino acids, vitamins A, B1, B2, B3, C and D, minerals iron, magnesium, copper, zinc, sodium, potassium, calcium, several glucosinolates, 20 free fatty acids, and unique compounds known as *Macaenes and Macamides.*

2. Maca is an adaptogen. Adaptogens are very uncommon plants (any other example is ginseng) that improve the bodily body's kingdom of resistance to illnesses via physiological and emotional health enhancements. Adaptogens have a normalizing effect, i.e., Counteracting or preventing disturbances to homeostasis brought about by stressors. Moreover, they offer a broad

range of therapeutic effects without causing any major side effects.

3. Maca balances hormones in women and men. One of the very great things about peruvian maca root is that it isn't always "gender specific" and works equally well for both women and men in terms of achieving hormone balance. Sustained and accelerated energy is a result of a positive balance of hormones.

Which Maca Is Best for Energy Boosting

From my own experience Red Maca is great because it's the highest in phytonutrient content material of all maca colors. Black Maca is also very good and for men it's probably the best as it also has been shown to boost libido and sperm count in males.

CHAPTER 5

What Is Black Maca?

Black Maca is called Lepidium Meyenii in Latin. It is a tuber that was originally grown in the highlands of the Andes Mountain in Peru, principally close to the Lake Junin region. While the crop was only adapted to the cooler mountainous region, it was traded drastically throughout the ancient Incan Empire with the highlands indigenous peoples buying and trading Black Maca root for other lowland stale crop such as corn and quinoa.

For thousands of generations, then, the Andean peoples have recognized the several health benefits related to the Black Maca plant. Similar in size to a large radish or small turnip, this root vegetable also resembles a type of white carrot. The small green leaves never grow more than 20 cm of the ground, making this a unique plant in that most of the growth takes place underground.

The actual roots of the maca plant, which are the edible part of the plant, range in size and shape and can be spherical, rectangular and even triangular. Moreover, the color of the root can range from a gold or cream color, to darker shades of reds, purples and blacks. Black maca is by far the most common and the most recognized by the outside world for its health benefits.

Understanding The 3 Colors of Maca

If you were to visit a Maca farm in Peru at some point of the annual harvest you would see that Maca roots grow in 3 ranges of colors:

- White to Yellow roots are called Cream Maca

- Light Pink to Dark Purple roots are called Red Maca

44

- Light Gray to Dark Gray roots are called Black
  Maca

Of the three colors Black Maca is the rarest.   Cream
Maca makes up about 60% of the harvest, Red Maca
about 25% and Black Maca about 15%.   Note: Black
Maca is the one in the middle of the picture to the right.

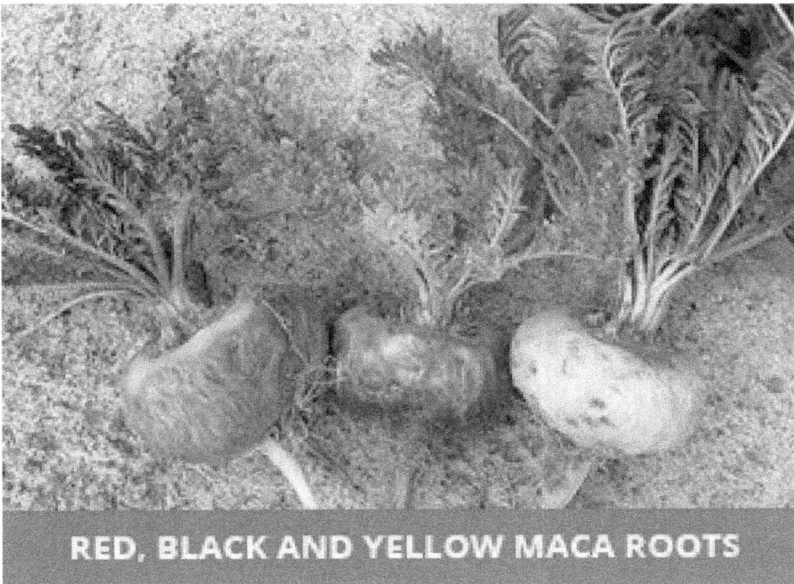

RED, BLACK AND YELLOW MACA ROOTS

The three Maca colors are all from the same species and
sub-species of plant and traditionally were lumped
together when Maca powder was produced.   However

starting about 15 years ago, the roots began to be separated when making powder because research suggested each color to have some different properties and uses.

What Studies Have Been Done on Black Maca?

In 2010 a review paper published by Institute of Plant, Animal and Agroecosystem Sciences in Zurich; Switzerland concluded that different colors of Maca root certainly do have specific health promoting properties. This review became stimulated by several other research papers focused on both Red and Black Maca in the middle 2000s.

Here Is A Summary Of What Research Has Uncover On Black Maca So Far

- In a study from 2009 at a Peruvian University, Black Maca turned out to be the best Maca for increasing sperm production motility and volume as well as for increasing libido.

- In 2011 two different research, one from China and one from Peru found that Black Maca helped laboratory mice improve their memory and concentration competencies.

- In 2010 a team of 6 researchers suggested that Red and Black Maca were found to be the best at improving and protecting bone structure especially in mice who had their ovaries removed.

- And in 2006 a Peruvian team discovered that while all Maca contributed favorably to lowering depression, Black Maca also improved the learning and concentration skills of laboratory mice.

Other ongoing research has recommended that Black Maca works barely better than the other colors for muscle building and endurance purposes.

Who Ought to Take Black Maca?

Based at the research we cite above; Black Maca is sometimes considered as "Men's Maca." I often receive questions asking if women can also take it.   Even as Black Maca does work better for male fertility and libido than other Maca colors, women can and do take it frequently. This is due to the fact Maca, regardless of color, does not contain any hormones.   Instead, it stimulates the body to achieve healthy hormone stability.

Black Maca, raw and gelatinized, is my second best choice of maca and my experience combined with the research above leads me to recommend it for:

- Men wishing to increase their fertility (women should try Red Maca for fertility)

- Women and men wishing to enhance or increase their libido

- Athletes, both women and men, seeking out for more stamina and energy

- Absolutely everyone trying to improve memory, concentration and focus abilities with Maca

- All people taking Maca to improve their bone strength and density (Red Maca has also been shown to be useful for this motive)

A Few Things to Look for When Buying Black Maca

It is always important to consider the source quality and freshness of any Maca product you purchase because ultimately this will determine how effective it is. Here are a few pointers to help you make the best choice:

- ***Purchase only Peruvian Maca*** - the best Maca comes from the high Andes in Peru. There are now Chinese Organizations or Companies trying to grow Maca and producing fake Maca in labs. I recommend avoiding any Maca from China.

- ***Insist on organic*** - Maca can and is grown organically and traditionally without the use of pesticides and chemicals. (Note that the research above were all performed exclusively with organic Maca roots)

- ***Get the freshest*** - Maca is only harvested once a year, but has a shelf life of 2 years. Try and purchase Maca from the current year's harvest and make sure that it is comes in a container which completely seals out humidity, light and oxygen. This will preserve the freshness of the powder and get you better results.

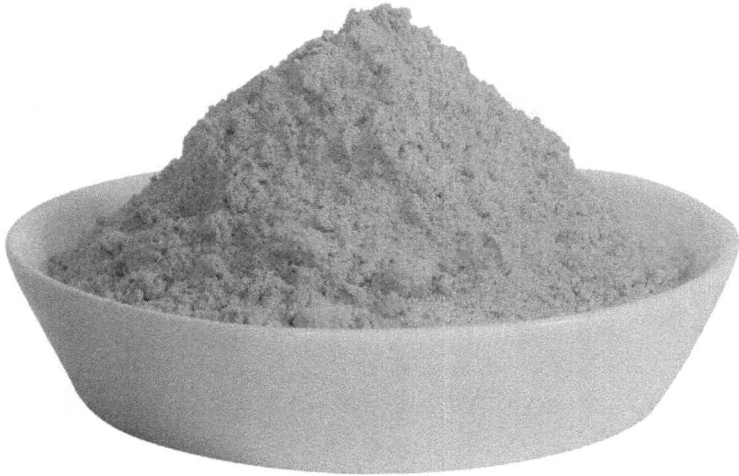

- ***GMO- Free -*** this is easy considering the fact that Peru has banned all GMO (genetically modified organisms) from all of its agriculture till 2021 (yippie!).

One final thing to keep in mind about Black Maca is that the powder will be only barely darker than Cream Maca. The reason for that is that Black Maca roots are something like a radish in that the color is predominately in the skin.

CHAPTER 6

8 Benefits of Black Maca

What exactly are the health benefits that the Incans knew of and what does modern day scientific investigation inform us about the advantages and medicinal properties of this unique plant? Below we look at eight of the most important health and dietary benefits of Black Maca.

1. High in Protein and Essential Vitamins

Even as many people take Black Maca for its health properties that we will explore below, it is actually one of the most overall nutritious foods on the market. One ounce of Black Maca powder will give you over 130% of your vitamin C, 4 grams of protein, and 85% of your everyday copper consumption. It is also a good source of other essential vitamins and minerals such as iron, potassium and manganese.

2. Libido Enhancer

Daily intake of black maca has additionally been demonstrated to boost sexual desire in both women and men. The improved fertility that supposedly comes with consuming black maca is most possibly because of the increased libido that comes with this unique plant. One latest research confirmed that black maca root does enhance the sex drive in healthy, middle age men.

3. Alleviate Signs of Menopause

Along with increasing the sex drive, black maca has also been proven to help relieve the worse signs and symptoms of menopause in women. While there are several symptoms related to menopause, one study found that black maca is mainly effective in helping to lessen hot flashes and irritability at night.

4. Increases Endurance

Many professional athletes, bodybuilders, and weight lifters have recently begun taking black maca dietary supplements due to the increased endurance that it gives in the course of extreme physical activity. Swimmers specifically have determined that regular consumption of black maca allow them to go longer and farther during training.

5. Protects from UV Radiation

Much has been written these days about the potential risks of immoderate utility of sunscreen which may in fact include several carcinogens. For those who are looking for more natural and safer alternative, black maca extract, while applied to the pores and skin can help to guard your body from the harmful UV rays of the sun.

6. Reduce Prostrate Size

The prostate gland causes all forms of problems in aging men. From difficulty with urinating to prostate cancer, many men worry about the problems that come with getting old. Regular consumption of black maca might thoroughly help to reduce the size of the prostate gland in men. Considering the fact that larger prostate glands can cause problems passing urine and probably cause most cancers, black maca consumption is encouraged in ageing men, not to say that it may also help induce sexual desire.

7. Enhance Memory

Regular consumption of black maca can also help to

improve your overall brain functioning. From helping children with learning disabilities to enhancing your long term memory, regular intake of this important root can be essential for maintaining a healthy, alert brain and memory.

8. Increase Fertility

Now not only does black maca root improve libido, there's also some evidence showing that black maca root may also enhance the sperm quality in men. For men who're having fertility issues, black maca can be an important addition to other varieties of fertility treatments.

Approaches To Consume Black Maca

Unless you stay in chilly, mountainous vicinity above 13,000 feet with confined amounts of sunlight, you probably won't have much good luck trying to grow your personal black maca. While black maca root can be consumed like any other root vegetable, most of the commercial black maca cultivation dries the root into powder form. Dried black maca root can last for several years while still keeping its nutritional and medicinal properties.

It is also possible to gelatinize maca root via gentle heat and pressure. This process separates the thick fibers from the rest of the root making it easier to devour. Most of the black maca root sold in pill form is available in gelatinized form. Although less common, you can also discover liquid extracts of black maca root as well.

CHAPTER 7

Pros Of Black Maca Powder and Dosage Information

By far, the most common way to eat black maca is in powdered form. As referred to above, the main benefits of ingesting black maca powder is that the hypocotyls which are in the root can be stored for several years without losing their medicinal and nutritional properties.

There are several different methods to take black maca powder depending on what you are using it for. However, most medical professionals endorse taking it as a dietary and medicinal supplement on a daily basis. Anywhere between 1 and 5 grams per day of black maca powder is the usual dosage.

Pros Of Black Maca Capsules and Dosage Information

Black maca can also be taken in pill form. For people who've weak digestive tracts, black maca tablets or pills will usually contain gelatinized forms of black maca root. This process removes the entire thick, hard to digest fibers from the plant and allows for less complicated digestion. A 500 mg tablet or pill can be taken once a day to begin with. In case you sense you want a more potent dose; you can take up to a gram in pill form safely.

The Best Way to Consume Black Maca

The best way and manner to consume black maca relies largely on your personal state of affairs and context. If you can get fresh black maca root, simply cooking up the root like a potato will offer you the most direct benefits. In case you pay a visit to Peru or a few other Andean countries, you may also be able of get your hands on bulk black maca flour that's genuinely dried and powdered black maca root which would be the best bang for your buck.

If you are looking for commercial products, powdered black maca is usually the preferred option due to the versatility it gives. With powdered black maca, you may mix it into shakes or smoothies to cover up the nutty taste that some people do not particularly enjoy.

Black Maca Side Effects

As a totally natural product, black maca has virtually no side effects. However, black maca is known to affect the hormone levels in human beings, so it ought to not be taken by other people who are on other chemical medications for hormone treatment. Moreover, people with high blood pressure need to also visit a medical professional earlier than taking black maca on a regular basis.

CHAPTER 8

WHAT IS RED MACA?

Red Maca (lepidium meyenii or lepidium peruvianum) is the second rarest of all varieties of maca, making up about 25% of the yearly harvest. It is sometimes referred to as pink or purple Maca, however is most generally known as "Red Maca." It grows in the regions and under similar contions as other more common types of Maca and yet has some unique properites that are quick making it the Maca of preference. During the last few years it has gain quite a bit of popularity and quite without a doubt, once we tried it 2 years ago, it has become our favourite variety not only because of the increased efficiency, but also because of the taste.

How is Red Maca Different?

If you were to visit a Maca farm, before the roots are made right into a powder, you'd quickly and without difficulty be able to tell the difference between Red Maca, Yellow/Cream Maca and Black Maca. As you can see from the images right here, every of the roots are of a special shade – and on this way they're named.

Even though all organically grown high quality Maca powders shares a nearly equal dietary profile, Red Maca has been shown, under phytonutrient analysis, to be higher in certain compounds that supports the body in antioxidant and antitumoral activity. It has been show amongst all Maca colors to contain somewhat higher levels of other pythonutrients which includes alkaloids, tannins, saponis and steroids.

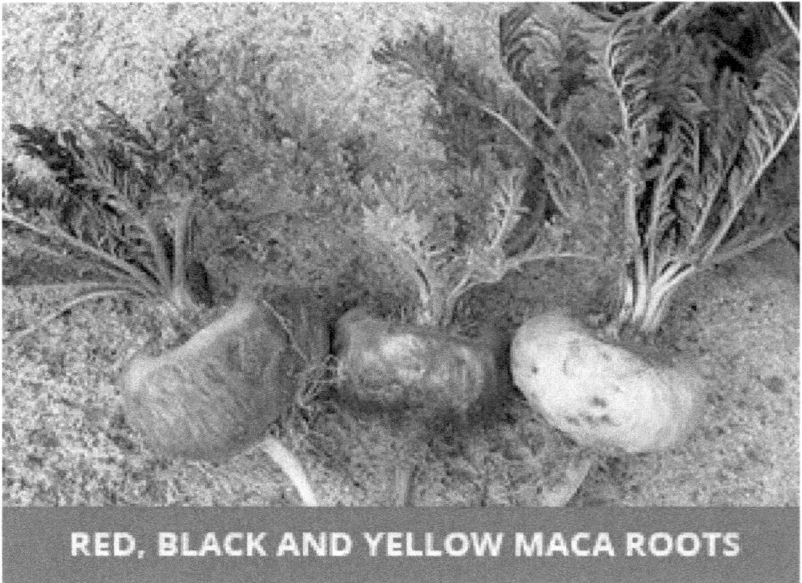
RED, BLACK AND YELLOW MACA ROOTS

Another substantial difference between Red Maca and Cream or Black Maca is the taste. The majority find the taste to be gentle and mild. We've found that to be true as well and might describe the taste as similar to a subtle caramel. One of my clients lately wrote me to allow me to know that her kids love Red Maca on their oatmeal in preference to sugar as it tastes so sweet!

What Studies Have Been Carried Out On Red Maca?

Interest in Maca amongst medical professionals is growing as are research studies. In terms of studies on Red Maca powder particularly, there are three main tremendous ones.

1. The most vital study done on Red Maca was published in the journal reproductive Biology and endocrinology 2005; 3:5. In it 8 medical researchers report that over the course of 42 days: "Red Maca however neither Yellow/Cream nor Black Maca reduced significantly ventral prostate size in rats." the studies also goes on to document that under pyhtochemical analysis for 7 RED-Webfunctional nutrient groups, "Highest peak were observed for Red Maca, intermediate values for Yellow/Cream Maca and low values for Black Maca."

2. In 2010 researchers from the Universidad Peruana, Lima published a study on the effects of Maca on bone structure in rats that had had their ovaries removed. The conclusion was that both "Red and Black Maca have protective effects on bone architecture in OVX rats without showing estrogenic effects on uterine weight."

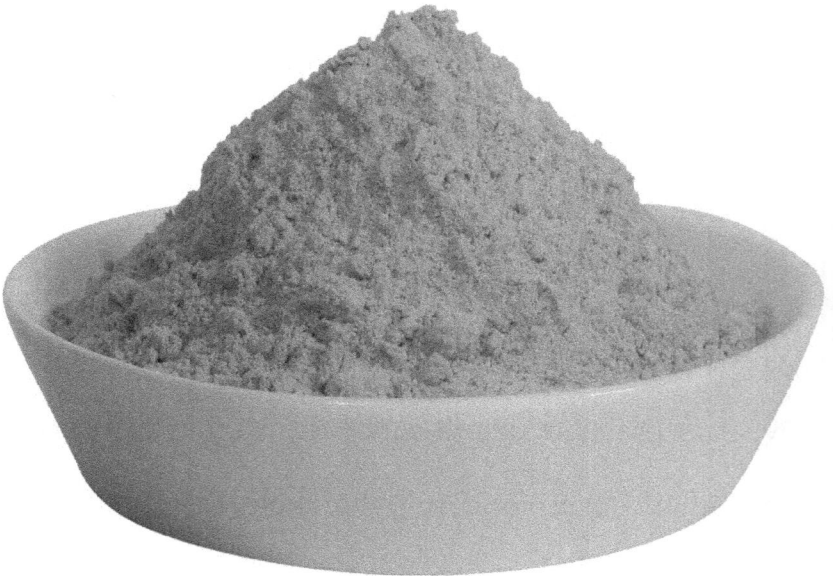

3. Finally another study from the same University in 2009 found that Black Maca to increase sperm production more than Yellow or Red Maca. The study

concluded that while Red Maca, like other Macas, had a favorable effect on energy, mood and sexual desire, it did little to increase the volume of sperm produced in comparison to Black or Yellow Maca.

How Can Red Maca Support Vibrant Health?

Red Maca, just like the Yellow/Cream and Black Maca can do all the following:

- Boost overall energy and vitality

- Balance hormones for both women and men – this can support with menopause, pimples, fertility, thyroid and other health problems associated with the endocrine system.

- Support a healthy libido and sex drive.

Similarly Red Maca mainly appears to be the best colors for:

- Prostate protection – most important for men and in particular men over 40

- Bone density – most important for women and children

Complete Dietary Breakdown of Red Maca

Sample length 100g:

Carbohydrates 62.6g, fats 0.82g, fiber 5.3g, protein 17.9g

Protein components (%): Albumins & Globulins 74, Glutelins 15.3, Prolamins 10.6, True protein 42.1

Vitamin & minerals (mg %): Ascorbic acid 3.52, Boron 12, Calcium 490, Iron 80, Magnesium 70, Niacin 43, Phosphorous 320, Potassium 113, Riboflavin 0.61, Sodium 20, Thiamine 0.42, Zinc 12.

Amino Acids: Alanine 63.1, Arginine 99.4, Asparatic Acid 91.7, Red Maca PowderGlutamatic Acid 156, Glycine 68.3, HO-Proline 26, Hystidine 21.9, Isoleucine

47.4, Leucine 91, Lysine 54.5 Methionine 28, Phenylalanine 55.3 Proline 0.5, Sarcosine 0.7, Serine 50.4, Threonine 33.1, Tyrosine 30.6, Valine 79.3

Final Thought on Red Maca - Raw Vs. Gelatinized

I love all kinds of Maca and have enjoyed the benefits of them for years. I like to use variety of Maca colors for myself and normally have Cream, Red and Black Maca on hand. That said, my favorite tasting Maca is Red Maca. I highly recommend it as it offers nearly all the advantages of the other forms of Maca with the exception of increasing sperm count.

Major marketers now sell Red Maca in both raw and gelatinized bureaucracy. For most people i recommend the raw product as all of it's nutrients are 100% intact. However, when you have a sensitive stomach or an issues with digesting starch you're better off getting the gelatinized product.

CHAPTER 9

WHAT IS YELLOW MACA?

Maca root powder is a loved a part of life in the high Andes. Yellow Maca is the most common of all colors, making up about 60% of the annual harvest. Ours is made from roots traditionally grown and harvested on an organic farming co-op in a remote pristine part of the Peruvian Andes. It is never heated above 106 degrees F in an effort to preserve nutrients at maximum levels. Yellow Maca has been the most researched of all three maca colors.

- Yellow Maca is nutrient dense with 60% carbohydrates, 12 crucial minerals, 10 vitamins, over 40 fatty and amino acids and 4 unique glucosinolates – a true superfood.

- Used for over 2000 years as a nutritionally dense food to promote endurance, vitality, fertility and libido in populations living at very high elevations.

- Grown in the Andes at elevations above 14000 feet and in extreme cold, wind and sunlight, Maca is the world's highest growing crop

- As Yellow Maca is the most common Maca it's also the least expensive.

Yellow Maca Root Powder Is:

- Certified Organic

- GMO Free

- Fair Trade

- Grown traditionally with respect for the land - near Junin, Peru

- Sun dried, carefully processed and packaged

without delay

- 100% Raw and Vegan

- Contain Only Yellow Maca Root Powder

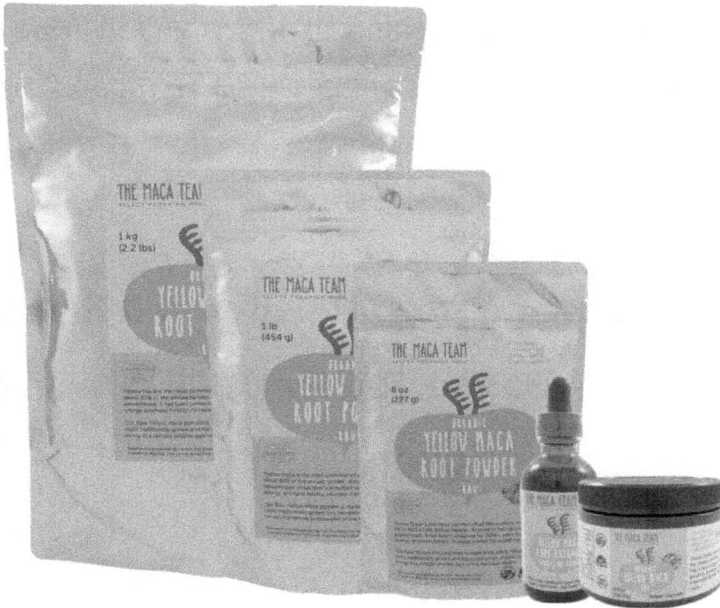

Yellow Maca Powder Is A Great Way To Begin With Maca.

To this point loads of researches, all available publicly in the pubmed database, has found it to be useful for energy building, fertile, hormone stability or balance, mental awareness and more. Yellow Maca is certainly a nutritional powerhouse, containing nearly all essential amino acids and free fatty acids, substantial levels of vitamins A, B1, B2, B3, and C, minerals iron, magnesium, zinc and calcium, a high concentration of bio-available protein and nutrients unique to Maca called *Macaenes* and *Macamides*. Maca is also an *"Adaptogen,"* or rare form of plant that is thought to elevate the overall life force energy of those who eat it.

Cream Maca Root Powder In 3 Sizes: (Servings Based Totally On 3 Tsp Or 9 g Every Day)

- 8 ounces (25 servings)
- 16 oz (50 servings)
- 1 kg - 35 ounces (111 servings) - exceptional price!

In vegan capsules

- 750 mg every, 2 hundred ct (28 servings)

And in glycerine based liquid extracts

2 fl oz (59ml)

CHAPTER 10

Maca Root Benefits

Maca root is a tuber that is also referred to as *"Peruvian Ginseng."* according to Mountain Rose Herbs:

Natives of this area ate it raw, cooked or boiled leading to its implementation as an everyday staple. The rough terrain of this vicinity made it difficult to cultivate food, so most of the communities' diet was based upon wild collected material. Maca resembles a radish and is actually a close relative. The growing conditions are very specific and it will only thrive in the glaciated slopes of the Andes with a prime elevation of 12,000 to 15,000 toes above sea level.

Maca has gained a reputation for helping balance hormones and reverse hypothyroidism. It is an endocrine adaptogen, meaning that it does not contain any hormones, but rather it includes the nutrients necessary to support normal hormone production.

It has also been used as a way to increase fertility (and i can vouch for this personally!). It is evidently "high in minerals (calcium, potassium, iron, magnesium, phosphorus, and zinc), sterols (6 found), up to twenty essential fatty acids, lipids, fiber, carbohydrates, protein, and amino acids."

Maca is regularly recommended to those with adrenal fatigue because it nourishes them and reduces stress hormones. It's specially regarded for its benefits in balancing hormones.

Maca root helps balance our hormones and due to an over abundances of environmental estrogens, most people's hormones are a bit out of whack. Maca stimulates and nourishes the hypothalamus and pituitary glands which are the "master glands" of the body. These glands clearly regulate the other glands, so whilst in balance they can convey stability to the adrenal, thyroid, pancreas, ovarian and testicular glands.

Maca root has been proven to be useful for all kinds of hormonal problems including PMS, menopause, and hot flashes. It is also a fertility enhancer and is best known for improving libido and sexual characteristic, particularly in men. For that reason, it's earned the nickname *"nature's Viagra."*

1. Rich in Antioxidants

Maca root acts as a natural antioxidant, boosting levels of antioxidants like glutathione and superoxide dismutase within the body. Antioxidants help neutralize harmful free radicals, fighting off chronic ailment and preventing damage to cells.

One test-tube study in 2014 tested that polysaccharides extracted from maca had high antioxidant interest and were powerful in fighting free radical damage.

An animal study in the Czech Republic even found that administering a concentrated dose of maca to rats now not only improved their antioxidant status, but also significantly decreased cholesterol levels and triglycerides in the liver and reduced blood sugar, helping prevent the development of chronic disease. Meanwhile, another test-tube study showed that the antioxidant content of maca leaf extract may even be of help to protect against neurological harm or damage.

RICH IN ANTIOXIDANTS

• Acts as a natural antioxidant

• Boosts levels of glutathione & SOD, among other antioxidants

• May help fight chronic disease & neurological damage

Improving your antioxidant status can be beneficial for stopping conditions like heart disorder, most cancers and diabetes with the aid of preventing oxidative stress and cell damage. However, despite these promising outcomes, more studies are needed to understand how the antioxidants in maca root may have an effect on people.

2. Enhances Energy, Mood and Memory

Individuals who frequently use maca powder report that it makes them feel more awake, energized and driven, often quite fast after beginning to use it. Plus, maca can help increase energy without giving you the "jitters" or a sense of shakiness like *high level of caffeine can*.

Clinical trials have proven that maca may also definitely impact energy and stamina. Maintaining positive energy levels can also help improve mood, and a few early studies have even found that maca may also lessen symptoms of depression.

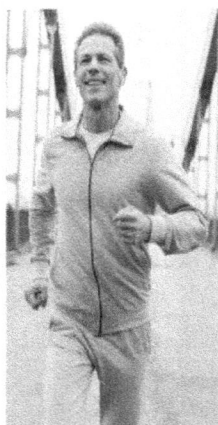

ENHANCES ENERGY,
MOOD & MEMORY

• Clinical trials have shown that maca may positively impact energy & stamina

• Animal studies have also found that maca root benefits memory & focus

• Some early studies have even found that maca may reduce symptoms of depression

It remains uncertain exactly how maca will increase energy levels; however, it's believed to help prevent spikes and crashes in blood sugar and maintain adrenal health, which regulates mood and energy throughout the day. Keeping energy levels up might also help prevent weight gain as well.

Numerous researches have also discovered that maca root benefits memory and focus. In fact, two animal research studies in 2011 showed that black maca was able to enhance memory impairment in mice, probably thanks to its high antioxidant content.

3. Improves Female Sexual Health

A couple of research has showed that maca benefits female sexual health through numerous different mechanisms.

Maca root may be able to enhance sexual dysfunction

and increase sex drive in women. One study looked at the results of maca root on post-menopausal women with sexual dysfunction caused by the use of antidepressants. Compared to a placebo, maca root is able to significantly improve sexual function. Any study had similar findings, reporting that maca was well-tolerated and capable of improve libido and sexual function.

A study in 2008 also found that maca root benefits both psychological symptoms and sexual function in post-menopausal women. In fact, maca was able to lessen menopause-associated depression and anxiety after six weeks of treatment.

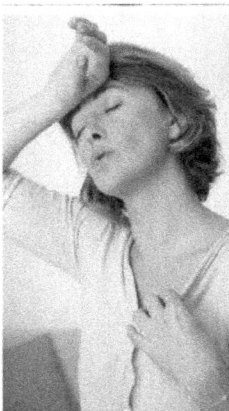

IMPROVES FEMALE
SEXUAL HEALTH   3

• May be able to improve sexual
dysfunction and boost sex drive in women

• Benefits psychological symptoms & sexual
function in post-menopausal women

• Helps balance female sex hormones &
alleviate symptoms of menopause

Maca is also able to balance female sex hormones and has even been proven to alleviate symptoms of menopause.

Balancing hormone levels is vital to many aspects of reproductive health and can help lessen signs and symptoms like infertility, weight gain and bloating.

4. Balances Estrogen Levels

Estrogen is the primary female sex hormone responsible for regulating the reproductive system. An imbalance in this crucial hormone can cause a slew of signs and symptoms starting from bloating to irregular menstrual periods and mood swings. Estrogen levels that are too high or low can also make it hard for a woman to ovulate and become pregnant.

Maca root can help stabilizes hormone levels and control the amount of estrogen within the body. One study published in the *International Journal of Biomedical Science* gave 34 early post-menopausal women a pill containing either maca or a placebo twice each day for 4 months. Not only did maca help balance hormone levels, however it also relieved signs of menopause, inclusive of night sweats and warm flashes, and even accelerated bone density.

In addition to reducing symptoms of menopause, regulating estrogen levels may also help with enhancing reproductive health and fertility and decreasing symptoms related to situations like ***polycystic ovary syndrome*** (PCOS), such as excess hair growth, weight gain and acne.

BALANCES ESTROGEN LEVELS

4

• Can help balance hormone levels & control the amount of estrogen in the body

• Can relieve menopause symptoms, such as night sweats & hot flashes

• May help bone density, decrease PCOS symptoms & improve reproductive health

5. Boosts Male Fertility

So what about maca root for men? Research show that maca powder benefits male sexual health and fertility as well.

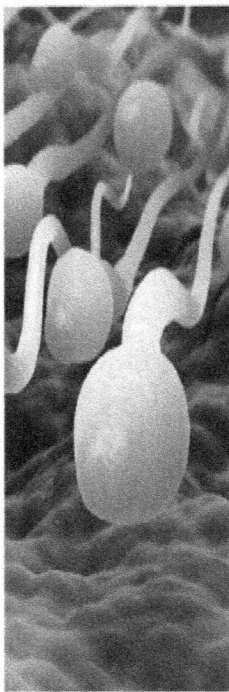

BOOSTS MALE FERTILITY

5

• Studies show that maca powder benefits male sexual health & fertility

• Can increase sexual desire

• May improve sperm quality & motility, two important factors when it comes to male infertility

One study out of Peru found that supplementing with maca for eight weeks increased sexual preference in men. Meanwhile, another study in 2001 showed that maca helped improve sperm quality and motility, two essential factors when it comes to male infertility.

Maca may also benefit sexual dysfunction as well. A 2010 review summarized the results of 4 clinical trials evaluating the effects of maca on libido and suggested that two of the studies showed an improvement in sexual dysfunction and sexual desire in both women and men. However, the alternative two trials did not find a positive end result, so further research is still needed.

CHAPTER 11

7 Things To Understand About Correct Maca Dosage

1. Maca is a food – initially, it's important to take into account that natural maca powder, whether gelatinized or raw is a meals. It comes from a turnip like root high in the Andes mountains and has been eaten for thousands of years by people and animals indigenous to the vicinity. Maca is in contrast to other foods, though, in that it's a true nutritional powerhouse and an adaptogen.

2. You can't overdose, but… – from my own experience it's pretty much impossible to take too much of Maca. (Since it's a food and not a drug, herb or supplement). That said, some people report increased coronary heart rate and nervous energy when they take too much. That's

why you need to start with a conservative amount and work your way up slowly.

3. You have to consider your body weight - whilst you're starting with Maca, you need to consider how much you weigh as an important factor in figuring out your dosage. The dosage levels i suggest beneath are for those who weigh 160 pounds (75 KG). Bigger people can generally take more. Smaller people need to start with a smaller quantity.

4. You should also consider your general health and age – after factoring in your weight, also reflect on your overall level of health and your age. A 30-year-old athlete can start taking a higher Maca dosage than a 75-year-old retiree. The younger and healthier you are the more you can begin with.

5. Maca affects different people differently – even factoring in age, health and body weight, it's important to

remember the fact that Maca has different effects on different people. No two bodies are exactly alike and for the reason that Maca is an adaptogen it will act in your body to support what your body needs to balance – particularly in terms of your hormonal system.

6. You may regulate quantities as needed – one thing that we do often hear is to adjust the amount of Maca we take depending on how much energy we need, or how long way we've come along in our health goals. Sometimes we'll even forestall taking Maca for some days, whilst we feel like a break – more of that during a minute.

7. Therapeutic Maca dosage is different than general health dosage – one very last consideration is that recommended dosages of Maca for therapeutic purpose are usually higher than for general health. For example if you are taking Maca in particular to help with fertility, you may need to boost your intake over time.

My General Maca Dosage Recommendations - Powder - Capsules - Extracts

These dosage levels are primarily based on a forty-year-old with generally good health and weighing 160 lbs. If you weigh more or less adjust the dosage accordingly. *Note:* 1 measuring teaspoon of Maca powder weighs 3 grams.

Raw Maca – all colors together with Red Maca, Black Maca and Yellow Maca

Daily Recommendations – 3-9 grams (1-3 teaspoons) or 2-8 capsules

Raw Premium Maca

Daily Recommendations – 3-6 grams (1-2 teaspoons) or 2-8 capsules

Gelatinized Maca – all colors such as Red, Black and

Yellow Maca (note: despite the fact that Gelatinized Maca is more concentrated, I will advise the equal amount to make up for the fact that some nutrients were destroyed by heating it).

Daily Recommendations – 3-9 grams (1-3 teaspoons) or 2-8 capsules

Gelatinized Premium Maca

Daily Recommendations – 3-6 grams (1-2 teaspoons) or 2-8 tablets

Maca Extracts

Daily Recommendations – 2-4 droppersful (1/4-1/2 teaspoon)

CHAPTER 12

Where To Find and How To Use Maca Root

At this point in time, you're probably wondering: "where can i buy maca?"

Thanks to its growing popularity, maca is broadly available at health stores, pharmacies and even on-line retailer. It can also be found in pill, liquid, powder or extract form. All forms are thought to be equally beneficial, however it's best to buy maca from a quality harvester that guarantees its 100 percent pure maca root powder. Ideally, you should also look for a variety this is raw and organic.

Additionally, maca is categorized based on the color of its roots and is most commonly yellow, black or red. All colors of maca have similar benefits, despite the fact that precise maca types and colors are thought to be more beneficial for certain medical conditions.

Maca tends to have an earthy, barely nutty taste with a hint of butterscotch that works specifically well when added to oatmeal or cereal. The taste may vary based on the type of maca, with black maca being a bit more sour and cream-colored roots having an even sweeter taste. Maca powder can be easily added to smoothies and drinks or mixed into recipes.

Keep in mind that most people prefer not to microwave or warmness their maca powder at high temperatures because the heating method may decrease some of the nutrients.

In the Andes Mountain, locals may consume as much as a pound of dried or fresh maca root daily. Most people supplement with somewhere between one gram to 20 grams daily in powder form.

Despite the fact that there is no official recommended maca powder dosage, it's best to start out with about one tablespoon (in powder shape) daily and work your way up to two to three tablespoons spread throughout the day. Due to the fact maca is known for increasing energy and stamina, many people like to take it before exercising to get a burst of extra energy.

Side Effects

Dietary supplements and drugs affect the body in a similar manner. They can enhance health but sometimes at a price. Some herbs, kava as an example, may cause organ damage, however the side effects associated to Maca appear less intense. An experiment described in the 2008 volume of "Food and Chemical Toxicology" assessed the protection of Lepidium consumption in patients experiencing symptoms of diabetes. Participants acquired either Maca or Placebo for 60 days. This treatment increased diastolic blood pressure. It also increased aspartate transaminase, a caution sign for tissue damage. Both changes were small, and their medical relevance remains unclear. Yet, the general public is urged to await more safety information before taking maca.

About the Author

Dionisia Onio is an Health Researcher from Italy who has developed a series of fabulous and highly effective healthful strategies. She applies her knowledge and astonishing perception to analyze the background and underlying causes of various diseases and health related problems affecting people in the world and then designs individualized and totally effective strategies to attain the desired results in solving human related problem with diseases.

Acknowledgments

The Glory of this book success goes to God Almighty and my beautiful Family, Fans, Readers & well-wishers, Customers and Friends for their endless support and encouragements.

www.ingramcontent.com/pod-product-compliance
Lightning Source LLC
Chambersburg PA
CBHW031904200326
41597CB00012B/532